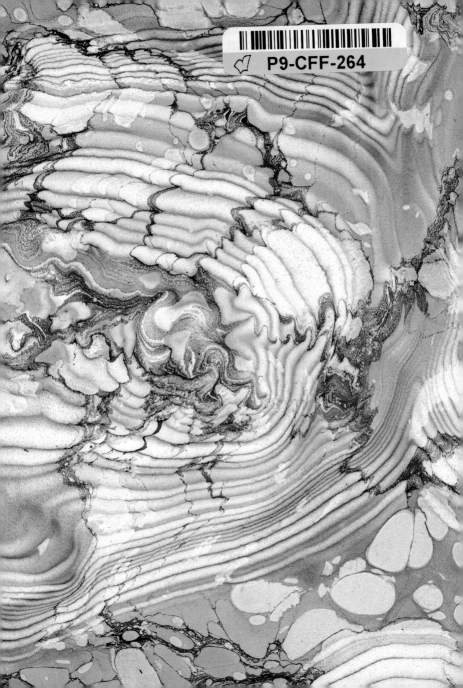

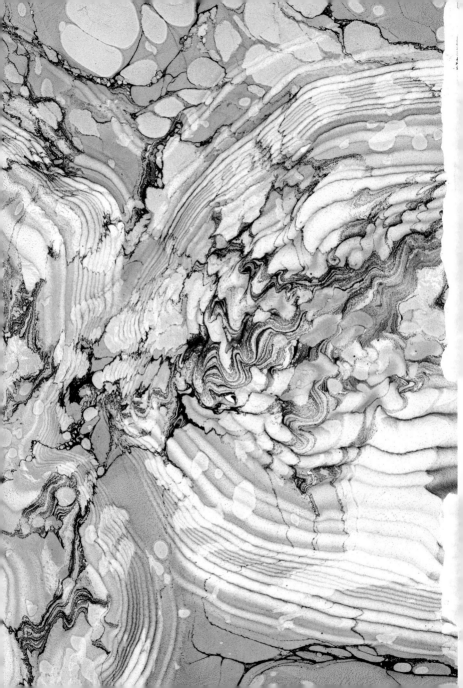

The Scented Bath

THE
SCENTED
BATH

A GIFT OF LUXURY FROM NATURE'S GARDEN

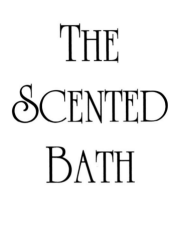

MARIBETH RIGGS

MARBLED PAPERS BY WENDY ADDISON

VIKING
STUDIO
BOOKS

Note: This book contains recipes using dried herbs, essential oils, and other ingredients that, when mixed properly and used externally are perfectly safe. However, certain of the contents may cause an allergic reaction in some individuals, so reasonable care in the preparation and use of these baths is advised.

VIKING STUDIO BOOKS

Published by the Penguin Group
Viking Penguin, a division of Penguin Books USA Inc., 375 Hudson Street, New York, New York 10014, U.S.A.
Penguin Books Ltd, 27 Wrights Lane, London W8 5TZ, England
Penguin Books Australia Ltd, Ringwood, Victoria, Australia
Penguin Books Canada Ltd, 2801 John Street, Markham, Ontario, Canada L3R 1B4
Penguin Books (N.Z.) Ltd, 182–190 Wairau Road, Auckland 10, New Zealand

Penguin Books Ltd, Registered Offices: Harmondsworth, Middlesex, England

First published in 1991 by Viking Penguin, a division of Penguin Books USA Inc.

1   3   5   7   9   10   8   6   4   2

Library of Congress Cataloging in Publication Data
Riggs, Maribeth.
The scented bath : a gift of luxury from nature's garden / baths by Maribeth Riggs : marbled papers by Wendy Addison.
p.   cm.
Includes 20 theme-bath recipes.
ISBN 0-670-83172-7
1. Aromatherapy. 2. Essences and essential oils—therapeutic use.
3. Erotic art. I. Addison, Wendy. II. Title.
RM666.A68R54 1991
615'.321—dc20

Printed in Japan.

Marble specimens from Granite and Marble World Trade, San Francisco, California.
Marble photography by Kirk Amyx, San Francisco, California.

Contents

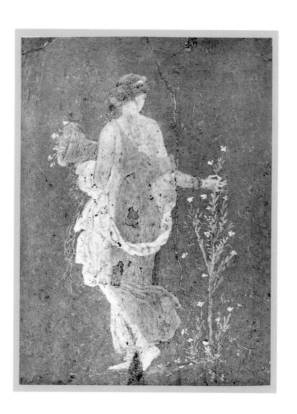

INTRODUCTION

The luxurious delight of aromatic bathing has been with us for centuries. In the magnificent bathhouses of ancient Rome, costly oils and fragrant unguents were applied before, during, and after the bath; and in parts of the world where bathing with water was not always practical, aromatics alone were employed to cleanse, condition, and perfume the skin. The refreshing and antibacterial qualities of the essential oils were prized by these ancient bathers. Now, by blending modern scented oils and skin-soothing bath products, you can experience and enjoy enchanting bathing rituals from around the world.

Aromatic bathing can affect you in many exquisite ways. Fragrances that are pleasing to the nose can also alter the mood. Combinations of natural essences can be formulated to have particular effects upon the body and mind. For example, eucalyptus, rosemary, wisteria, and citrus are light essences that stimulate and uplift. Patchouli, jasmine, ylang-ylang, and sandalwood are heavy essences that soothe and sedate. Lavender, sage, rose, and ginger are middle essences that act as a balancing link between aromas that stimulate and aromas that sedate. It is the combination of these aromas that makes each of the scented baths in this book a truly special event.

THE SCENTED BATH contains twenty theme-bath recipes designed to create a specific bathing experience for you. You may select a bath to lift your mood, to comfort your body, or to transform your appearance. If you wish to unwind after a hectic day, for example, the *Kashmir Breeze* or *Rose Milk Silk Bath* will pamper you with their intoxicating oils of rare flowers. If you've just finished a vigorous workout and would like to cool down, the *Bath Named Desire* or the *Lemon Zest Float* will make you feel delightfully refreshed. If your spirits need a gentle lift, charm yourself with the *Scottish Spring* or *Marjoram Sauvage Plunge*. Sore muscles are quickly soothed in the *Baden-Baden* or the *Summer Seashore Soak*. Get in touch with your innermost self during the *Full Moon Bath* or the *Japanese Bath Ceremony*. And experience a true rejuvenation of body and mind by indulging in the *Clan of the Cave Bear Spa* or the *Fountain of Youth*.

There's a bath for every mood, every fantasy, every occasion. When the inspiration strikes, transport yourself to an *Evening in Paris*, or to a *Fantasy Island Hot Spring*, or to a *Hawaiian Jungle Paradise*. Whichever bath you select, you will emerge realizing that you have just given yourself a precious gift of luxury from nature's garden.

Bath bags are a wonderful and simple way to release the oils of dried herbs into your bath. To make your own bath bag, choose a thin, rough-textured, brightly colored washcloth. Fold it in half and sew up the long edge and one short edge to form a pouch. Turn the pouch inside out and you have your bath bag, ready to fill with dried herbs and tie closed with a piece of ribbon.

While you run your bath, let the herbs contained in the bag soak in the hot water. After the bath is run, allow the bath bag to float in the water, and squeeze it repeatedly to infuse the water with the herbs. If you wish, you may use the bath bag to scrub and stimulate your skin. To reuse the bath bag, untie the ribbon, discard the wet herbs, and turn it inside out to dry until you are ready to use it again.

There are now many charming stores that supply the luxury bath products included in THE SCENTED BATH. Here, you can find the scented soaps, essential oils, loofa mitts, bath bags, talcum powders, scented splashes, dried herbs, and other delights you will be enjoying. If you do not have a bath store nearby, consult the *Bath Luxuries Shopping Guide* on page 61 for a full range of products from around the world that can be ordered by mail or phone.

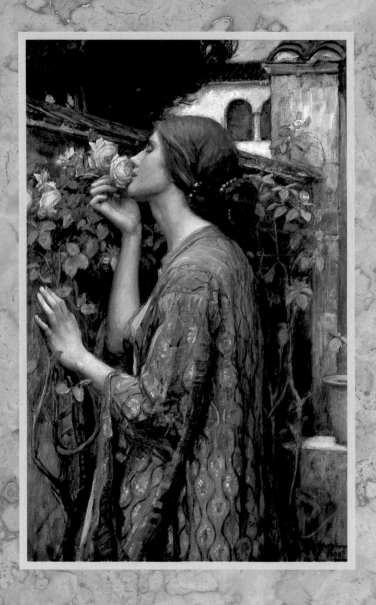

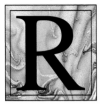

OSE MILK SILK BATH

Happiness lies in the fulfillment of the spirit through the body.
— Cyril Connolly

Your bath is a place of quiet, a private world where you can gently put aside the demands of your everyday life. Once you are alone, let the burdens of the day lift and empty your mind of all your concerns. Visualize a rose petal floating in a tranquil pool, and allow your thoughts to drift. Slip into a silken robe and prepare yourself for a beautiful bathing experience — the Rose Milk Silk Bath.

> *Two Cups of Powdered Milk*
> *One Packet (About One-Half Cup) of Colloidal Oatmeal*
> *Ten Drops of Oil of Rose Geranium*
> *Two Drops of Oil of Peppermint*
> *One-Half Cup of Rose Water*
> *One Perfect Rose in Full Bloom*

Draw your bath and slowly add the Powdered Milk and the Colloidal Oatmeal, swirling the bathwater as they dissolve. The water will now be opaque, as silky-feeling as the wrap you are wearing. The scent of the oatmeal will be light and sweet. Before you turn off the tap, add the Oil of Rose Geranium and the Oil of Peppermint, again gently swirling the water to combine.

When your bath is full, the temperature ideal, and the surface calm, add the Rose Water. Dip your hands into the water. It will feel silky soft, and the scent of roses will drift up like a fresh bouquet, surrounding you with its exquisite aroma. Now, remove the petals from your Perfect Rose in Full Bloom and drop them one by one onto the surface of the water.

Slip off your robe and ease yourself into the tub. Lie back, close your eyes, and take a deep breath. Let your body become weightless, your arms float to the surface, and your fingers relax and open. The scent of rose has long been known to release inhibitions. Certainly this is a perfect opportunity to let your imagination run free. Surrender to your fantasies.

O, my luve is like a red, red rose,
That's newly sprung in June.
O my luve is like the melodie,
That's sweetly played in tune.

As fair art thou, my bonie lass,
So deep in luve am I,
And I will luve thee still, my dear,
Till a' the seas gang dry.

Till a' the seas gang dry, my dear,
And the rocks melt wi' the sun!
And I will luve thee still, my dear,
While the sands o' life shall run.

And fare thee weel, my only luve,
And fare thee weel awhile!
And I will come again, my luve,
Though it were ten thousand mile!

— *Robert Burns*

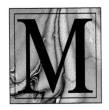

ARJORAM SAUVAGE PLUNGE

Paradise is a center whither the souls of all men are proceeding, each sect in its particular road.
— *Napoleon Bonaparte*

The Marjoram Sauvage Plunge is a bracing boost, best taken in the morning. Men love to soak in this earthy, green-scented bath — there is nothing timid about the exhilarating eucalyptus aroma with its citrus and cinnamon undertones. You will be washed with a buoyant feeling of optimism, and your naturally sunny disposition will awaken to greet the new day!

> *One Ounce of Dried Marjoram Leaves*
> *Ten Drops of Oil of Eucalyptus*
> *Cotton Bath Bag (see page 9)*
> *Ten Drops of Oil of Bergamot*
> *Ten Drops of Oil of Lavender*
> *Three Drops of Oil of Cinnamon*
> *Eucalyptus-Scented Soap*

Place the Dried Marjoram Leaves in a bowl and add the Oil of Eucalyptus, stirring the mixture thoroughly with a spoon. After the ingredients have been combined, crush the leaves with your hands and fill the Cotton Bath Bag about two-thirds full. Tie the top of the pouch closed. Run an extra-hot bath and toss in the bath bag. As the tub fills, squeeze the bag to release its herbal essence. The water will turn a rich golden color. While the bath bag soaks, make yourself a cup of Earl Grey tea, stirring in one drop of the Oil of Bergamot. Accompany your plunge with music that soars, like your spirit — Vivaldi, or Bach's Brandenburg Concertos.

Before you get into the tub, run the cool water to adjust the temperature and add the remaining Oil of Bergamot, the Oil of Lavender, and the Oil of Cinnamon, swirling the water gently so that the oils are well combined.

Immerse yourself quickly in the water and feel your mood lift like a dew-drenched flower seeking the radiance of the morning sun. Try to experience each ingredient in your bath: the stimulating aroma of the eucalyptus; the light, refreshing scent of bergamot; the sharp, subtle fragrance of lavender; and the brisk whisper of spicy cinnamon.

As you rub your body with the Eucalyptus-Scented Soap, imagine yourself plunging into the sparkling water of a glacial lake. You will step out of the Marjoram Sauvage Plunge feeling invigorated, and ready for a day of good cheer.

I

The word of the sun to the sky,
The word of the wind to the sea,
The word of the moon to the night,
What may it be?

II

The sense to the flower of the fly,
The sense of the bird to the tree,
The sense to the cloud of the light,
Who can tell me?

III

The song of the fields to the kye,
The song of the lime to the bee,
The song of the depth to the height,
Who knows all three?

— *Algernon Charles Swinburne*

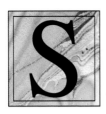

UMMER SEASHORE SOAK

*My God, a moment of bliss. Why, isn't that enough
for a whole lifetime?*
— *Fyodor Mikhailovich Dostoyevsky*

Spring, fall, and winter all offer up their unique pleasures, but it is the lazy, long, sun-drenched days of summer that make us feel young and alive again. Even during the dreariest months you can instantly shake off those winter doldrums and take off to the warmest, most carefree season of all. Just lower yourself into the Summer Seashore Soak and let your senses recall the feel, the smell, even the sounds of summer by the sea.

Two Ounces of Dried Kombu Seaweed
Two Cups of Sea Salt
One Cup of Baking Soda
Fifteen Drops of Oil of Rosemary
Sea Sponge
Lemon-Scented Soap

Begin by combining the Dried Kombu Seaweed (available at health food stores) with two quarts of water in a pot with a tight-fitting lid. Let the solution come to a boil, and then simmer slowly for about twenty minutes. While you are waiting you might like to treat yourself to a facial by lifting off the lid and letting that warm sea-smelling steam escape and envelop you. Close your eyes and take a couple of deep breaths.

After your steam facial, splash icy cold water on your face, and gently pat it dry. Now, put on some soothing music, or perhaps an environmental recording of the subtle rhythms of the sea. Fall into your favorite chair and roll your head slowly — first to the right, then to the left, and repeat. This simple relaxing exercise will release some of the tension that can gather in your neck, even on the calmest of days.

The kombu solution is ready, and you can draw your bath. Strain and discard the herb — the seaweed tea will have a gelatinous quality and a tawny ocean-bottom hue. Pour the hot liquid into your bath. Add the Sea Salt and the Baking Soda, slowly pouring them into the water still running from the tap. Gently swirl the bathwater to dissolve them.

Just before you turn off the tap, add the Oil of Rosemary to the bath and swirl the water to combine. Dim the lights and light a rosemary-scented candle. Rosemary is the herb of pleasant remembrances. Float the Sea Sponge in your bath and use the Lemon-Scented Soap to add a tangy zest.

Now it is time to close your eyes and let the water lap gently around you. Cast your mind back to the curl of a wave gathering force, to walks on the beach at dusk, to the feel of salty sea water tingling and caressing your toes as it spreads fingers of foam along the wet sand. As the heady aroma of rosemary rises around you, the herbal ocean tea will make your skin feel as if it is being tickled all over by a soft ocean breeze.

To me the sea is a continual miracle,
The fishes that swim — the rocks — the motions of
*   the waves — the ships with men in them,*
What stranger miracles are there?

— Walt Whitman

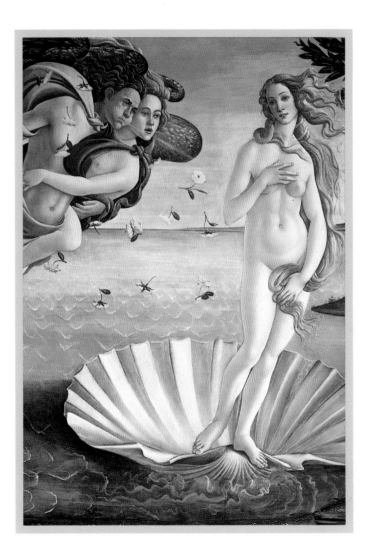

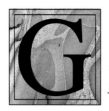

GONE WITH THE WIND BATH

Whether a pretty woman grants or withholds her favors, she always likes to be asked for them.
— *Ovid*

Courtly love, softly spoken words whispered in a secret moment, the sweet anticipation of a fancy dress ball — this is the romantic spell of the Old South, where the ladies are beautiful, the men are gentlemen, the way of life is a slow unfolding of social grace and pleasure. Imagine the gleaming white columns of plantation mansions, the sweep of manicured emerald-green lawns, and rows of live-oak trees hung with Spanish moss reaching to the ground. Wrap yourself in a soft, rose-covered robe and find a spirited waltz to play softly in the background. You might just believe that there are real musicians playing beneath your veranda, readying for the waltzes and Virginia reels you'll be dancing later in the evening. Find a perfectly ripe peach that you can enjoy while you bathe, and prepare your Gone with the Wind Bath.

> *Ten Drops of Oil of Jasmine*
> *Ten Drops of Oil of Wisteria*
> *One-Half Cup of Rose Water*
> *Carnation-Scented Soap*
> *Florida Water*

Run the bathwater to a comfortably warm temperature, and just before turning off the tap, add the Oil of Jasmine, the Oil of Wisteria, and the Rose Water. Swirl the bathwater gently to combine.

A heady bouquet of flowery scents will fill your bathroom. The essence of wisteria is especially intriguing. It is believed to clear the head and stimulate the mind, and it combines beautifully with the enchanting scent of rose water. Your senses will awaken to the intoxicating fragrance of night-blooming flowers.

Before you emerge, lather your skin with the Carnation-Scented Soap. Now rinse, step out, and wrap in a fluffy, white cotton towel. Before dressing, be sure to splash the Florida Water all over. You will feel cool and light, and the co-mingling of scents will give you the sought-after aura of a true flower of the South.

> *There was a land of Cavaliers and*
> *Cotton Fields called the Old South...*
>
> *Here in this pretty world*
> *Gallantry took its last bow...*
>
> *Here was the last ever to be seen*
> *of Knights and their Ladies Fair,*
> *Of Master and of Slave...*
>
> *Look for it only in books, for it*
> *is no more than a dream remembered,*
> *a Civilization gone with the wind...*

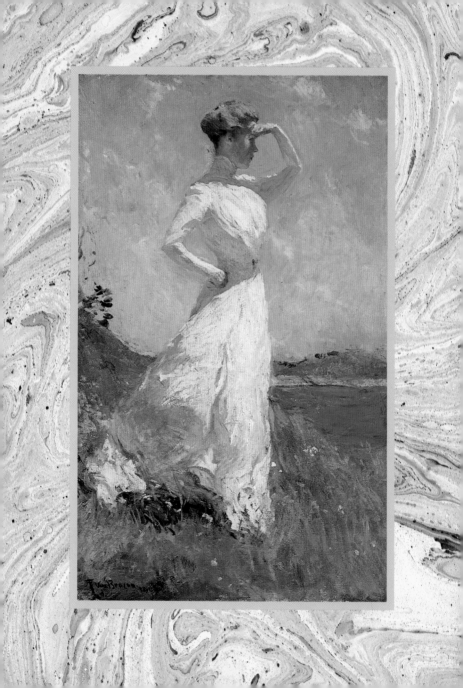

ALPINE MEADOW HONEY BATH

The influence of fine scenery, the presence of mountains, appeases our irritations and elevates our friendships.
— *Ralph Waldo Emerson*

Picture the Swiss Alps in spring, soaring snowcapped peaks emerging from the top of the world. The air is crisp, thin, and clear. In the shade you feel chilled, but beyond the shadow of the majestic trees you're warmed by a sun burning high in a cloudless, azure sky. You come upon an open but secluded meadow, filled with dancing wildflowers. Gentle bees gather their nectar for honey. A pale blue pool of water reflects the perfect sky. Capture the moment and relax in the Alpine Meadow Honey Bath.

> *Two Cups of Skim Milk Powder*
> *One-Half Cup of Honey*
> *Ten Drops of Oil of Lavender*
> *Ten Drops of Oil of Orange Blossom*
> *Pure Castille Soap*

Enjoy this bath on a weekend afternoon, when the sun is still streaming through the open bathroom window. Pour a tall, cold glass of mineral water and place it near the bathtub. Select lilting flute or rhythmic acoustic guitar music to play, and light a beeswax candle to enhance the bath's scent of honey and flowers.

As you run the water, add the Skim Milk Powder and the Honey, agitating the bathwater to dissolve and combine the ingredients. The water will take on a milky blue tint and a soft, silky feel. Just before you turn off the tap, add the Oil of Lavender and the Oil of Orange Blossom, and gently swirl the bathwater once more.

Now, slide into this perfectly prepared pool of pleasure. Allow the delicate aroma of orange blossoms to conjure up sunny spring days and cool mountain breezes. The bracing scent of lavender will tone your skin, leaving it tight and clean, as though sun kissed from a day in the clear Alpine air. Use the Pure Castille Soap and remember to sip your mineral water, to refresh yourself from the inside out.

The year's at the spring
And the day's at the morn;
Morning's at seven;
The hillside's dew-pearled;
The lark's on the wing;
The snail's on the thorn:
God's in his heaven —
All's right with the world!

— Robert Browning

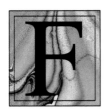 ULL MOON BATH

The power that holds the sky's majesty wins our worship.
— *Aeschylus*

As dusk melts into night and the full moon rises slowly to shed its silver light in an indigo sky, a magic moment occurs — your senses are heightened and the wisdom of the universe seems within reach. The full moon is a time of peak vitality, a time when your intuition and instincts are most sharply focused. The Full Moon Bath is designed to enhance your inner powers and delight your senses. Surrender yourself to the lunar forces.

> *Two Cups of Sea Salt*
> *Six Drops of Oil of Wintergreen*
> *Six Drops of Oil of Bayberry*
> *Six Drops of Oil of Ambergris*
> *Six Drops of Oil of Sage*

While running your bath, add the Sea Salt and the Oil of Wintergreen, the Oil of Bayberry, the Oil of Ambergris, and the Oil of Sage. Gently swirl the water until the salt is dissolved. Dim the overhead lights and light a tall white candle at the edge of the tub. The flickering light will cast a reflection that shimmers like the moon on a calm sea. The celestial sound of delicate flute music and a cup of warm chamomile tea are the ideal accompaniments to your full-moon experience.

Sit back in the bath, close your eyes, and inhale the deep, rich aroma of each of these lunar essences. Let the wintergreen sweep you away to a silent pine forest, where the needles are coated with crystalline snow. The scent of bayberry will fill you with a wonderful sense of well-being. The essence of sage will amplify the mood, while the heady fragrance of ambergris will continue to give pleasure for many hours.

Linger in your moonlit bath for as long as you like. Close your eyes. Feel the water lap around you and let your inner tides rise and fall until you feel rejuvenated and optimistic about the month ahead. Take this bath only during the full moon, so that at the beginning of each lunar cycle, the fragrances will refresh your mind and you will build, bath by bath, a reflective bridge into your future.

She walks in beauty, like the night
   Of cloudless climes and starry skies;
And all that's best of dark and bright
   Meet in her aspect and her eyes:
Thus mellowed to that tender light
   Which heaven to gaudy day denies.

One shade the more, one ray the less,
   Had half impaired the nameless grace
Which waves in every raven tress,
   Or softly lightens o'er her face;
Where thoughts serenely sweet express
   How pure, how dear their dwelling place.

And on that cheek, and o'er that brow,
   So soft, so calm, yet eloquent,
The smiles that win, the tints that glow,
   But tell of days in goodness spent,
A mind at peace with all below,
   A heart whose love is innocent!

— George Gordon, Lord Byron

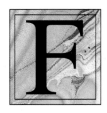

FOUNTAIN OF YOUTH

Vitality shows in not only the ability to persist but the ability to start over.

— F. Scott Fitzgerald

Recall the time when your life seemed to stretch out endlessly in front of you. Feel your youth, your energy, your enthusiasm, and optimism. Remember when anything was possible, when any future, any dream could come true? It's time to be young and spirited again, with ageless, firm skin and resilient, shiny hair. Let the Fountain of Youth restore and renew you.

One Cup of Aloe Vera Gel
Ten Drops of Oil of Rosemary
Ten Drops of Oil of Sweet Pea
Na-PCA Spray

Draw a comfortably warm, not-too-hot bath. As the water is running, add the Aloe Vera Gel, swirling the water well so that the gel is completely integrated with the bathwater. Aloe vera gel is available at health food stores, and will make the water in your bath feel soft and smooth. While the water is still running, add the Oil of Rosemary and the Oil of Sweet Pea, and stir with your hand until they are well combined.

Immerse yourself completely. You will relax in the Fountain of Youth for at least one-half hour. Put your head back and saturate your hair. As you soak, wet your hair often and allow the moisture-binding properties of the water to work their magic.

Notice how the aloe vera keeps your skin cool and nourished as it works with the bathwater's heat. Rosemary has long been known to add suppleness and tautness to the skin. Queen Elizabeth of Bohemia attributed her beautiful skin to the rosemary water that she used as a daily facial tonic. The scent of rosemary, combined with the vibrant green scent of sweet pea, brings forth a refreshing, rejuvenating essence of springtime that will linger on your skin.

After you've shed many years during your soak in the youth serum bath, towel off and complete your de-aging experience. Spray the Na-PCA on your face, throat, hair, and all over your body. Na-PCA Spray (sodium pyrrolidone carboxylic acid) is available at health food stores. It is a naturally occurring organic sugar that attracts and holds plumping moisture to your skin and hair, making it feel firm and young again.

> *Crabbed age and youth cannot live together:*
> *Youth is full of pleasance, age is full of care;*
> *Youth like summer morn, age like winter weather;*
> *Youth like summer brave, age like winter bare.*
> *Youth is full of sport, age's breath is short;*
> *Youth is nimble, age is lame;*
> *Youth is hot and bold, age is weak and cold;*
> *Youth is wild, and age is tame.*
> *Age, I do abhor thee; youth, I do adore thee.*
>
> — *William Shakespeare*

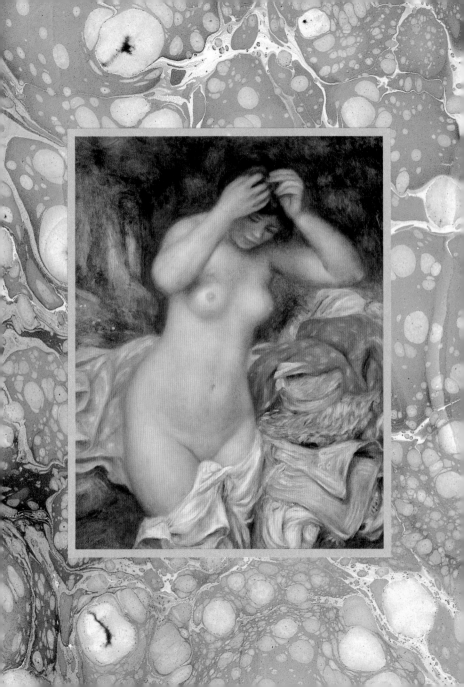

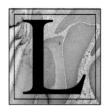

LEMON ZEST FLOAT

Running to the window, he opened it, and put out his head. No fog, no mist: clear, bright, jovial, stirring, cold; cold, piping for the blood to dance to; golden sunlight; heavenly sky; sweet fresh air; merry bells. Oh, glorious! Glorious!

— Charles Dickens

Perfection is beginning your day with a half-an-hour vitality float in an invigorating lemon-scented cloud. This pre-breakfast rejuvenator will clear the mental cobwebs from the sleepy night before and elevate your spirits for the day ahead. Enjoy the Lemon Zest Float with a half of a lemon squeezed into a glass of pure spring water — sweetened if you wish — to tone and cleanse you from within as well.

> *Twenty Drops of Oil of Lemon*
> *Ten Drops of Oil of Verbena*
> *One-Third Cup of Foaming Milk Bath*

Run your bath to your favorite temperature. When it is only one-fourth full, add the Oil of Lemon and the Oil of Verbena, and stir with your hand to combine them. Immediately pour the Foaming Milk Bath into the most turbulent part of the water. It will begin to foam into billowing clouds of bubbles as the tub continues to fill.

Milk baths give the water a rich feeling and impart silky smoothness to your skin. There is a wide variety of foaming milk bath formulas available at bath stores. Select one with a neutral scent. Soap is unnecessary, for the foaming milk bath will bubble your skin clean.

Throughout the ages, the spirited scent of lemon has been associated with robust health and freshness. Its buoyant aroma elevates the mood and invigorates the mind. The scent of verbena stimulates the circulation, giving your complexion a rosy, radiant glow. As you lie back and close your eyes, your feelings of lightness and floating will be enhanced. Imagine yourself drifting, floating ever higher. How high you go and for how long is, of course, up to you.

> Earth has not anything to show more fair:
> Dull would he be of soul who could pass by
> A sight so touching in its majesty:
> This City now doth, like a garment, wear
> The beauty of the morning; silent, bare,
> Ships, towers, domes, theatres, and temples lie
> Open unto the fields, and to the sky;
> All bright and glittering in the smokeless air.
> Never did sun more beautifully steep
> In his first splendour, valley, rock, or hill;
> Ne'er saw I, never felt, a calm so deep!

> — William Wordsworth

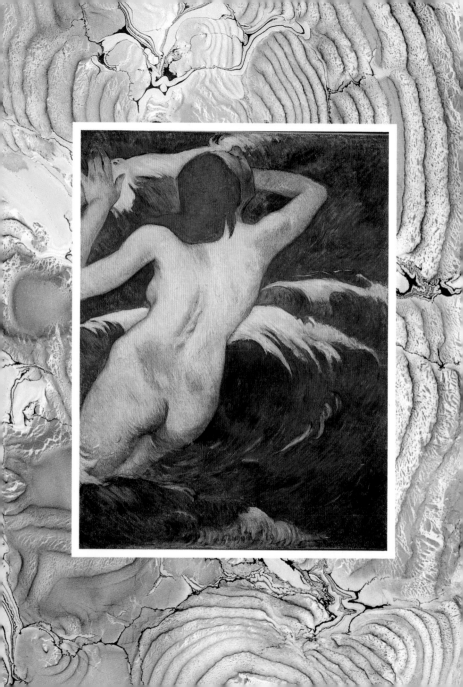

FANTASY ISLAND HOT SPRING

Some desire is necessary to keep life in motion, and he whose real wants are supplied must admit those of fancy.
—*Samuel Johnson*

Time out for luxury — welcome to a bath rite extraordinaire — the Fantasy Island Hot Spring. Patchouli, ylang-ylang, ginger, and cloves — even the names of these exotic essential oils can excite the senses with anticipated pleasure. This sensual bath, created from the tropics' most treasured plants, will transform your boudoir into an island paradise.

Fix your favorite tropical beverage — Piña Colada, Mai Tai, or the sparkling juices of mango or guava. Now, cut an unpeeled orange into six slices. Insert four cloves into each slice and place them on the edge of the tub. Later, you'll let the slices of orange float in the bath with you. Turn on some reggae or calypso music and, without spilling your drink, dance your way in the general direction of your Fantasy Island Hot Spring.

> *One Whole Orange*
> *Twenty-four Whole Cloves*
> *Five Drops of Oil of Patchouli*
> *Seven Drops of Oil of Ginger*
> *Three Drops of Oil of Clove*
> *Ten Drops of Oil of Ylang-Ylang*
> *Cocoa Butter*
> *Gardenia-Scented Soap*
> *Loofa Mitt*

Run a warm bath. When it is almost full, add the Oil of Patchouli, the Oil of Ginger, the Oil of Clove, and the Oil of Ylang-Ylang. Turn off the tap and float the clove-spiked orange slices on the surface.

Now, turn on your imagination, and while the pink sun slips behind the lush green hills, lower your sun-kissed body into the Fantasy Island Hot Spring, letting the gentle bubbling spring water surround you. The rich essence of the patchouli is frequently used in potions to attract love. The stimulating fragrance of ginger adds a hot sensation to the water. The scent of cloves is both exciting and comforting, and will leave a pleasant tingling on your skin long after your bath is done. The ylang-ylang flower gives a voluptuous, sweet scent to your bath. Be careful with the ylang-ylang, however — it is commonly believed that the oil is a powerful aphrodisiac.

Use the Gardenia-Scented Soap and scrub yourself lightly with the Loofa Mitt until your skin tingles. After you leave the bath, but while still wet, rub your warm skin with the Cocoa Butter. Your bathing experience will stay with you all day as you head back to the mainland feeling refreshed, alive, and open to the adventures ahead.

Here first she bathes, and round her body pours
Soft oils of fragrance and ambrosial showers,
The winds, perfumed, the balmy gale conveys
Through heaven, through earth, and all the aerial ways.

— Homer

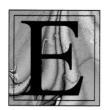

VENING IN PARIS

Settle down in Paris then. There are no mountains that I know of, and the only lake is the Bois de Boulogne, and not particularly blue. But there is everything else: plenty of pictures and churches, no end of celebrated men, and several beautiful women.

— *Henry James*

Paris! The City of Lights and glamorous nights, the place where the endless pursuit of beauty and style are a way of life. A discreet tapping at the door of your suite in the George V, and then a liveried waiter enters, bearing a lavishly appointed tray with an iced Daum champagne flute, a split of Veuve Clicquot, and one proud red rose in a pearl-white Limoges vase. You sweep into the *salon de bain*, the train of your Dior crepe de chine bath wrap swirling about your ankles, and your Evening in Paris has begun.

> *Ten Drops of Oil of Musk*
> *Ten Drops of Oil of Gardenia*
> *Musk-Scented Soap*
> *Gardenia-Scented Talcum Powder*

Run your bath to a comfortably warm temperature, and just before turning off the tap add the Oil of Musk and the Oil of Gardenia. Agitate the water with your fingers to carefully combine the oils. Glide into the lusciously aromatic water. The marriage of these two heady floral scents is a near perfect one, simulating the long-lasting strength and authenticity of the costliest French perfumes. The Oil of Musk contributes a full-bodied base note that develops differently on every woman's skin to create a heavenly signature scent. The Oil of Gardenia vibrates like a high note, floating sweetly in the air that surrounds you. Lather yourself all over with the Musk-Scented Soap to punctuate the moment.

After a glorious twenty minutes you will feel, look, and smell gorgeous. The grand finale — a light dusting with the Gardenia-Scented Talcum Powder and a coy dab of musk behind each knee.

Ah, happy, happy boughs! that cannot shed
  Your leaves, nor ever bid the Spring adieu;
And, happy melodist, unwearièd,
  For ever piping songs for ever new;
More happy love! more happy, happy love!
  For ever warm and still to be enjoy'd,
    For ever panting, and for ever young;
All breathing human passion far above,
  That leaves a heart high-sorrowful and cloy'd,
    A burning forehead, and a parching tongue.

— John Keats

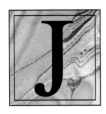

JAPANESE BATH CEREMONY

Blossoms are scattered by the wind and the wind cares nothing, but the blossoms of the heart no wind can touch.

— *Yoshida Kenko*

"My bath is a time of absolute quiet and meditation. An hour of stillness and calm in the storm of my day. I will linger in my bath so that when I am ready to leave it, my mood has been altered, my inner balance restored." This is your Japanese Bath Ceremony meditation.

> *One-Quarter Ounce of Dried Lemongrass*
> *One-Half Ounce of Fresh Ginger Pieces*
> *One Ounce of Dried Star Anise*
> *Twelve Drops of Oil of Pine Balsam*
> *Jasmine-Scented Soap*

Combine the Dried Lemongrass, the Fresh Ginger Pieces, and the Dried Star Anise with two quarts of water in a stainless steel pot. Cover with a tight-fitting lid. Bring the mixture to a boil and then let it simmer for five minutes. Steep the mixture for an additional fifteen minutes.

Meanwhile, slip into a silk kimono and burn a stick of sandalwood incense to set the mood. Sit, either on the floor or in a chair, with your back straight. Close your eyes, empty your mind, and picture yourself high on a mountaintop illuminated by sunset. Breathe deeply and slowly, and go into yourself. When you have been completely at peace for several moments, open your eyes. Remain still for five minutes more. Now that you are calm and centered, you are ready for the Japanese Bath Ceremony.

Begin running your bath. Strain the herbs from the steeped bath tea and add the solution to the bath. The water will become golden and slightly translucent. Just before you turn off the tap, add the Oil of Pine

Balsam. Place a bar of the Jasmine-Scented Soap tub-side. Your bathroom will now smell as though it has been transported to a wooded hillside in rustic Japan.

Lower yourself into the steaming bath. The balsam will bring a peaceful energy to lift and refresh your spirit, and the sweet spicy aroma of the dried herbs will linger on your skin for hours. After the calm of your meditation, the bath will penetrate and warm you, leaving you renewed and energized inside and out.

> *Blest, who can unconcernedly find*
> *Hours, days, and tears slide soft away,*
> *In health of body, peace of mind,*
> *Quiet by day,*
>
> *Sound sleep by night; study and ease*
> *Together mixed; sweet recreation;*
> *And innocence, which most does please*
> *with meditation.*
>
> — *Alexander Pope*

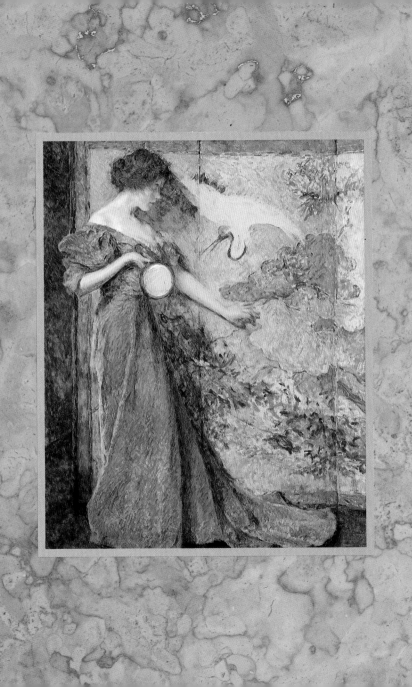

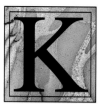

KASHMIR BREEZE

Safe upon the solid rock the ugly houses stand:
Come and see my shining palace built upon the sand!
— Edna St. Vincent Millay

East of the sun and west of the moon — the Kashmir Breeze, with its combination of precious ingredients, will allow you entrance to the fabled lands of floating flowers and Oriental opulence. Listen to the rustle of shimmering silks and the quiet metallic chime of temple bells, see a whirl of intense colors and patterns, and inhale the ever-present scent of exotic fragrances carried on a Himalayan breeze. Of these, there is none more prized than jasmine. In fact, oil of jasmine is nearly as expensive as gold. Its intoxicating scent and its mood-elevating effect are the ultimate gift of luxury from nature's garden.

> *Fifteen Drops of Oil of Jasmine*
> *Ten Drops of Oil of Ambergris*
> *Four Drops of Oil of Cinnamon*
> *Sandalwood-Scented Soap*

Make yourself a pot of sweetened Darjeeling tea, and add three whole cloves and a pinch of cinnamon. Let it cool tubside while you draw your bath. You might want to place a dish of plump dates nearby to munch as the pampered women of Kashmir do when they bathe recreationally. If you have a recording of Kitaro's *Silk Road*, play it softly.

Now, make certain to run bathwater that feels a bit hot at first, but of course not so hot that it's uncomfortable. Just before turning off the tap, add the Oil of Jasmine, the Oil of Ambergris, and the Oil of Cinnamon. Agitate the water to combine them well.

When you climb into the Kashmir Breeze bath you will surrender supremely to the wealth of fragrances. Like jasmine, ambergris is an especially rare and treasured essence, with an intoxicating, haunting aroma. The spicy-sweet scent of cinnamon adds a stimulating base note to this marvelous bath. Lather with the Sandalwood-Scented Soap to complete the aromatic mix and create the exotic enclave of an eastern paradise. Soak indulgently for at least twenty minutes, but stay submerged in this rich world for as long as your heart desires.

Here, Eve speaks to Adam.

With thee conversing I forget all time,
All seasons and their change, all please alike.
Sweet is the breath of morn, her rising sweet,
With charm of earliest birds; pleasant for the sun
When first on this delightful land he spreads
His orient beams, on herb, tree, fruit, and flower,
Glistring with dew; fragrant the fertile earth
After soft showers; and sweet the coming on
Of grateful evening mild, then silent night
With this her solemn bird and this fair moon,
And these the gems of heav'n, her starry train:
But neither breath of morn when she ascends
With charm of earliest birds, nor rising sun
On this delightful land, nor herb, fruit, flower,
Glistring with dew, nor fragrance after showers,
Nor grateful evening mild, nor silent night
With this her solemn bird, nor walk by moon,
Or glittering starlight without thee is sweet.

— John Milton

the Borax and the Sea Salt are completely dissolved.

Now it's time to claim your just reward. Slip into the tub and journey back to your earliest moments of sensation. Give your conscious mind a rest, and allow your unconscious feelings free rein. Soak for at least twenty minutes, and breathe deeply of the healing scents surrounding you.

The essential oils in the Baden-Baden bath are wonderful for restoring the body's vital energy and stimulating the respiratory system. When you are fully relaxed you may use the Loofa Mitt to invigorate your skin and circulation. Do not use soap with this bath. If you can, let your skin air dry before you dress.

Essential oils are wrung:
The attar from the rose
It is not expressed by suns alone,
It is the gift of screws.

The general rose decays;
But this, in lady's drawer,
Makes summer when the lady lies
In ceaseless rosemary.

— Emily Dickinson

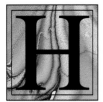# AWAIIAN JUNGLE PARADISE

*Zest is the secret of all beauty. There is no beauty
that is attractive without zest.*
— *Christian Dior*

Enter the jungle, a world where you can shed inhibitions and experience your most natural, most animal self. The pleasures you will seek are entirely physical. Your senses become more keen, more alive. You hear everything. You see everything. Give in to your most primitive desires as you experience the Hawaiian Jungle Paradise. Push the trailing vines aside and smell, taste, touch the humid, shadowy, fragrant atmosphere. There is no past or future, but only the moment and the powerful awareness of how alive you suddenly feel. Open yourself up to the wonder of it.

Before you run your bath, select a ripe, fragrant pineapple and slice it into pieces. Sprinkle shredded coconut over the slices and put them in easy reach of the tub. If you have glass or bamboo wind chimes, hang them near your bathroom window so that you can hear their mesmerizing sounds while you bathe.

> *One Ten-Ounce Can of Unsweetened Coconut Milk*
> *Ten Drops of Oil of Gardenia*
> *Ten Drops of Oil of Amber*

Run your bath and pour the Unsweetened Coconut Milk into the warm water, gently agitating until it is completely blended. Already you will feel the oil-rich coconut milk moisturizing the skin on your hand, while the tropical scent of coconut begins to fill the room. Add the Oil of Gardenia and the Oil of Amber, again swirling the bathwater until the oils are blended. Do not turn the tap off completely, but allow it to trickle slowly and softly during your bath.

Relax in your Hawaiian paradise and imagine the vibrant stillness of the jungle. You feel a oneness with all living things, and pause as they do, to listen to a soft, soothing, refreshing rain that sounds almost polite as it begins to fall.

The scent of amber is a rich, earthy one, suggesting the fecund growth of plant life around you. The gardenia is the essential flower of the tropics, enhancing this humid, dark green world with its compelling, mysterious intoxication. The oil in the coconut milk will cling to your skin. You may use a coconut-scented soap to emulsify it, or if you wish, use nothing at all and emerge from the tub with your skin glistening. No need to moisturize, just wrap up in a jungle print bath sheet and hold on to this untamed moment for as long as you can. Aloha.

> We grew in age — and love — together —
>   Roaming the forest, and the wild;
> My breast her shield in wintry weather —
>   And, when the friendly sunshine smil'd,
> And she would mark the opening skies,
> I saw no Heaven — but in her eyes.
>
> — Edgar Allan Poe

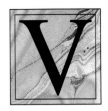

ICTORIAN POSY

"My love!" she cried, lifting her face and looking with frightened, gentle wonder of bliss. Was it all real? But his eyes were beautiful and soft and immune from stress or excitement, beautiful and smiling lightly to her, smiling with her. She hid her face on his shoulder, hiding before him, because he could see her so completely. She knew he loved her, and she was afraid, she was in a strange element, a new heaven round about her. She wished he were passionate, because in passion she was at home. But this was so still and frail, as peace is more frightening than force.

— *D.H. Lawrence*

Devoted masters of the art of scent mixing, the Victorians invented the science of aromatherapy and applied its uses in many marvelous ways. The Victorian Posy bath is a classic floral mélange that will enchant and brighten your hour of total luxury. To re-create the look of this bath, tie your hair up with a silk scarf or satin ribbon and place a bouquet of sweet peas or violets near the tub. If you're bathing at twilight, an arrangement of candles placed near a mirror will give even the smallest of bathrooms the spacious, grand feeling of Victorian elegance.

> *Six Drops of Oil of Rosemary*
> *Six Drops of Oil of Verbena*
> *Twelve Drops of Oil of Violet*
> *Six Drops of Oil of Rose Geranium*
> *Lavender-Scented Soap*
> *Rose-Scented Talcum Powder with an Oversized Puff*

While drawing your bath select your music. Brahms or Schumann played softly will allow you to travel back in time, inspiring the moods of the past. Just before you turn off the tap, add the Oil of Rosemary, the Oil of Verbena, the Oil of Violet, and the Oil of Rose Geranium, and swirl the bathwater gently with your fingers to combine.

Slip into your Victorian Posy bath, close your eyes, and let the beautifully scented steam work its magic. The famous French courtesan Ninon de Lenclos used the tangy green scent of rosemary in her secret beauty-bath formula. And the Victorians commonly believed that if verbena water was sprinkled in rooms where parties and other pleasures took place, guests would grow merrier and more carefree. Inhale the verbena's tantalizing lemon scent to feel the festive, romantic mood. The shy, ladylike scent of violets has long been associated with the virtues of simplicity, serenity, and peace, while the spicy, sexy scent of the rose geranium will inspire nostalgic thoughts of love.

When you are able, finally, to gather the will to lift yourself out of your luxury bath, wrap yourself in a fluffy towel until you are dry. Now, for the perfect Victorian finish, reach for your Oversized Puff and dust yourself all over with a cloud of the Rose-Scented Talcum Powder.

> *Let us have wine and women, mirth and laughter,*
> *Sermons and soda-water the day after.*
>
> — *George Gordon, Lord Byron*

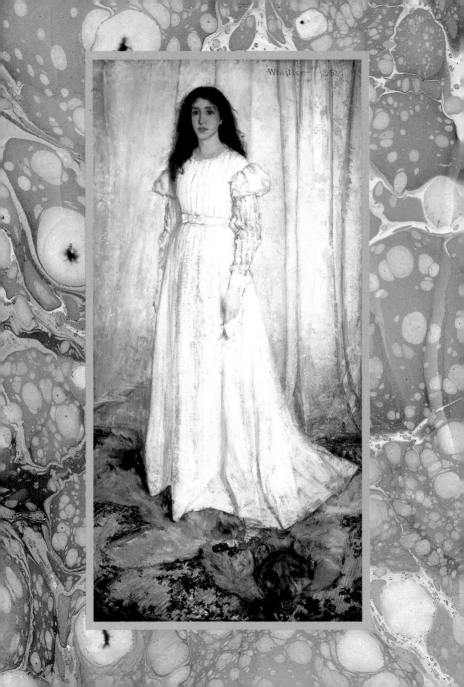

CLAN OF THE CAVE BEAR SPA

They looked at each other, baffled, in love and hate. All the warm salt water of the bathing pool and the shouting and splashing and laughing were only just sufficient to bring them together again.

— *William Golding*

The Clan of the Cave Bear Spa is a powerful, healthful ritual designed to purify the mind and body. Enter this prehistoric spa for a transforming retreat from the outside world. It will prepare you to embrace new situations with grace, and help you to accept life's challenges with courage and confidence. Once you have experienced its magical properties, you will return to this spirit-renewing ceremonial spa again and again.

> *One-Quarter Cup of Powdered French Clay*
> *Sage Smudge Stick*
> *Pine-Scented Soap*
> *Loofa Mitt*
> *Pumice Stone*

Warm your bathroom ahead of time so that you'll be comfortable outside the bathtub during the spa ritual. Prepare your Clan of the Cave Bear mud pack by mixing the Powdered French Clay with enough water to make a slightly runny paste. Take off your clothes, tie back your hair, and slather the clay on your face, neck, and upper chest.

While the clay is drying and drawing impurities from your skin, light the end of the Sage Smudge Stick and wave it in the air for a minute or two until the bathroom is redolent with the earthy scent of the burning herb. Smudge sticks, widely available at health food stores, are bundles of herbs tied tightly together so that when lit, the stick will smoke rather than burn. Sage was burned ritually by North American Indians to purify and cleanse the environment. It symbolizes the virtues of strength and wisdom, and the forces of the earth that can be summoned to counteract negative thoughts and influences.

Extinguish the smudge stick and fill the tub to the top with comfortably hot water. By now the clay will have dried on your skin, so you may climb in and submerge yourself. Splash water over your face and neck to soften the clay, and wash it off your skin with the Pine-Scented Soap. Pine has a powerful restorative scent that brings to mind positive, secure experiences. After ten minutes or so, scrub your skin with the Loofa Mitt to remove dry, dead cells and smooth your body all over. Continue to soak for another ten minutes or so.

Now, pull the plug and let the water drain out of the tub around you. While you are waiting, rub the Pumice Stone against the rough areas of skin on your elbows, feet, and hands — anywhere there are calluses to be smoothed away. When the tub is nearly empty, turn on the faucet to a cool temperature and squat in front of it, splashing water over yourself to rinse off.

You will now glow pink all over, purified from head to toe, mentally and physically. Rub your skin vigorously with a rough towel and let yourself air dry completely before you dress and emerge into the world, a more powerful entity.

> *Flower in the crannied wall,*
> *I pluck you out of the crannies,*
> *I hold you here, root and all, in my hand,*
> *Little flower — but if I could understand*
> *What you are, root and all, and all in all,*
> *I should know what God and man is.*
>
> — *Alfred, Lord Tennyson*

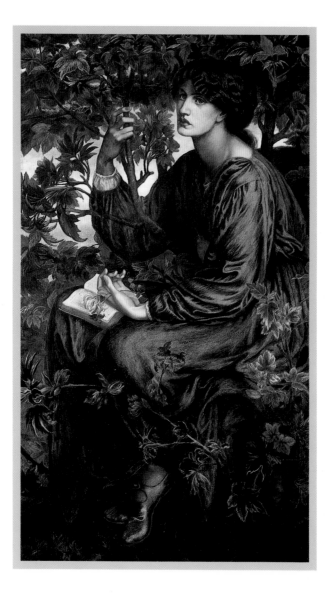

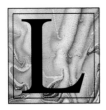

LADY OF THE WOODS

I got up early and bathed in the pond; that was a religious exercise, and one of the best things which I did. They say that characters were engraved on the bathing tub of King Tching-Thang to this effect: "Renew thyself completely each day; do it again and again, and again and forever again." I can understand that.

— Henry David Thoreau

Enter the sacred kingdom of a dark forest. Tall trees surround you, stretching for a bright blue sky. Shafts of emerald light angle their way through sylvan columns; the ground is dappled with sunlight. A woodland bouquet of pine and bark and young leaves rises up from the soft earth beneath your feet. You meander down a fern-lined path and come upon a clearing. There, sparkling through a curtain of dew-drenched fronds, lies a private pond, its surface a profusion of fragrant water lilies. Here, in this secret place, luxuriate in the warm waters of the Lady of the Woods bath.

> *One Ounce of Powdered Orris Root*
> *Twenty Drops of Oil of Amber*
> *Three Drops of Oil of Cedarwood*
> *One Ounce of Fresh or Dried Bay Leaves*
> *Ten Whole Cloves*
> *Cotton Bath Bag (see page 9)*
> *Sandalwood-Scented Soap*

In a bowl combine the Powdered Orris Root with the Oil of Amber and the Oil of Cedarwood. The orris root will remain powdery, even with the addition of the essential oils. Bruise and tear the Fresh or Dried Bay Leaves. Add the shredded leaves and the Whole Cloves to the powdered mixture, and evenly distribute them with your fingers throughout the orris root mixture. Fill the Cotton Bath Bag with the herbs.

Run a hot bath with the bath bag floating in the water. The naturally warming essences in the Lady of the Woods bath are released by the temperature of the bathwater. The powdery orris root will escape through the bath bag, making the water honey soft. If you wish, you can squeeze the bag to release more of its precious ingredients. The essential oils of amber and cedarwood will float to the top and moisturize your body as you submerge. Caress your skin with the spicy Sandalwood-Scented Soap. Its fragrance will linger long after you emerge from the tub.

Relax and rejoice in the woodsy, aromatic steam of the oils of amber and bay leaves. The Lady of the Woods bath will calm and center you, and the carefully combined scents will restore your harmony with nature. You'll feel as though you are caught in the tantalizing spell of an enchanted forest.

O hurry where by water among the trees
The delicate-stepping stag and his lady sigh,
When they have but looked upon their images —
Would none had ever loved but you and I!

O hurry to the ragged wood, for there
I will drive all those lovers out and cry —
O my share of the world, O yellow hair!
No one has ever loved but you and I!

— William Butler Yeats

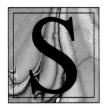

COTTISH SPRING

Happiness makes up in height for what it lacks in length.
— *Robert Frost*

Take a walk over the rugged and grand countryside of Scotland, at first in the bright sunshine and then in the gathering mist. When the afternoon turns colder and the mist swirls into rain, enjoy a highland hiatus — a steaming cup of tea and the soothing warmth of a Scottish Spring. The land of heather and tartans has long been known for its use of herbs for healing, cooking, and curative aquatic soaks.

As you prepare your bath, imagine yourself visiting a cozy stone cottage nestled high in the hills. You can see a flurry of clouds pass over a small village with cobblestone streets far below. As rain begins to fall softly, you hear the faraway sound of a sheep's insistent bleat. Settle yourself with a steaming pot of Earl Grey tea laced with milk and sugar.

> *One Packet (About One-Half Cup) of Colloidal Oatmeal*
> *Ten Drops of Oil of Lavender*
> *Five Drops of Oil of Rosemary*
> *Apple-Scented Soap*
> *Orange Water*

While your bathwater is running, add the Colloidal Oatmeal. It will cloud the water slightly and will give it body and softness. Swirl with your hands until the oatmeal is completely dispersed. Now add the Oil of Lavender and the Oil of Rosemary, swirling the water until the oils are well mixed.

Climb in, submerge, and inhale deeply. Lavender is a fragrance that blends wonderfully with rosemary, since the scent of lavender is pleasantly fresh and neutral. The combination gives the bath a green base, conjuring up for you the dewy highlands and low-lying heaths of Scotland. In time, you will come to associate these scents with feelings of inner warmth and coziness. Don't forget to sip your tea.

Just before you're done bathing, lather all over with Apple-Scented Soap for a tangy, exhilarating sensation. After you have dried off and noticed how the oatmeal has smoothed your skin, splash handfuls of the Orange Water all over. This delicate scent will complement the other light fragrances on your skin and make it feel like a Scottish wildflower welcoming the warmth of the sun on an early spring day.

To touch the cup with eager lips and taste, not drain it;
To woo and tempt and court a bliss — and not attain it;
To fondle and caress a joy, yet hold it lightly,
Lest it become necessity and cling too tightly;
To watch the sun set in the west without regretting;
To hail its advent in the east — the night forgetting;
To smother care in happiness and grief in laughter;
To hold the present close — not questioning hereafter;
To have enough to share — to know the joy of giving;
To thrill with all the sweets of life — is living.

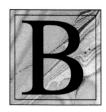

BATH NAMED DESIRE

*Only passions, great passions, can elevate the soul
to great things.*
— *Denis Diderot*

On summer evenings, when the hot air shimmers and your joie de vivre is evaporating, infuse the water in your bath with a tinglingly fresh sensation. In the nighttime world of gay nineties New Orleans, delightful scents defined a fancy lady's toilette — the perfume of the precious oils of magnolia and orange blossom wafted through the streets of the French Quarter, beckoning to the elegant gentleman the certain promise of beauty and romance.

To prepare for the Bath Named Desire, you will want to place two drops of the Oil of Peppermint into an ice-cube tray filled with water. Stir the oil so that it is well mixed and then allow time for the ice cubes to freeze solid. If you would like a mint julep to sip while you bathe, crush a few Peppermint Ice Cubes into your drink.

> *Four Drops of Oil of Peppermint*
> *One Tray of Peppermint Ice Cubes*
> *Ten to Fifteen Drops of Oil of Magnolia*
> *Ten Drops of Oil of Orange Blossom*

Run a hot bath. While the tub is filling, drop in the Oil of Magnolia, the Oil of Orange Blossom, and the remaining two drops of the Oil of Peppermint. Swirl the bathwater until the oils have been combined. Fill a bowl with the Peppermint Ice Cubes and put it at the side of the tub.

When the bath is full, climb in and lie back quietly until you are very warm indeed. Now, take an ice cube in each hand and slowly run the ice cubes over your body while you remain immersed. The ice will melt quickly, so reach for more until all the cubes are melted.

Now, relax and close your eyes and experience the exhilarating

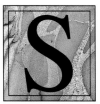

SWEET DREAMS BATH

Oh sleep! it is a gentle thing,
Beloved from pole to pole!
— Samuel Taylor Coleridge

The wonderful, languorous sensation of suspended animation just before you drift off to sleep is one of life's great pleasures. The feeling of absolute contentment when you are snuggled under warm covers, cozy and comfortable, is something to look forward to night after night. Anyone who needs a little coaxing to surrender to dreamtime will relish a soak in the Sweet Dreams Bath. Its sedative properties and soothing fragrances are guaranteed to bring a yawn to the lips of every restless night owl.

> *Cotton Bath Bag (page 9)*
> *One-Half Ounce of Dried Chamomile Flowers*
> *One-Half Ounce of Dried Rosebuds and Petals*
> *One-Half Ounce of Dried Basil Leaves*
> *Ten Drops of Oil of Lavender*
> *Five Drops of Oil of Bergamot*
> *Almond-Scented Soap*

Turn back the coverlet on your bed, plump up the pillows, and make your bedroom inviting for your return later on. Dim the lights and play soft, soothing music that has pleasant associations for you. Slip into a warm, comfortable robe.

Fill a Cotton Bath Bag with the three dried herbs and tie it securely. Begin to draw a bath, three-quarters full, with very hot water and immerse the bag while the water is running. Let the bag soak while you prepare a cup of chamomile tea. When you return to the bathroom, add cool water to reach your perfect bathing temperature and squeeze the bath bag repeatedly to release the herbal essences. Just before turning off the tap, add the Oil of Lavender and the Oil of Bergamot, and stir to combine them.

Lower yourself into your Sweet Dreams Bath. Lie back and place the bath bag behind your neck. Rest quietly and sip your tea for about twenty minutes. Then, finish your bath with a light body scrub: lather the bag with Almond-Scented Soap and massage your skin from the feet up.

Afterwards, bundle up in your favorite sleeping clothes, turn out the lights, climb into bed, and breathe deeply and evenly. Sweet dreams and good night!

Now sleeps the crimson petal, now the white,
Nor waves the cypress in the palace walk:
Nor winks the gold fin in the porphyry font.
The firefly wakens. Waken thou with me.

Now droops the milk-white peacock like a ghost,
And like a ghost she glimmers on to me.
Now lies the Earth all Danaë to the stars,
And all thy heart lies open unto me.

Now slides the silent meteor on, and leaves
A shining furrow, as thy thoughts in me.

Now folds the lily all her sweetness up,
And slips into the bosom of the lake;
So fold thyself, my dearest, thou, and slip
Into my bosom and be lost in me.

— Alfred, Lord Tennyson

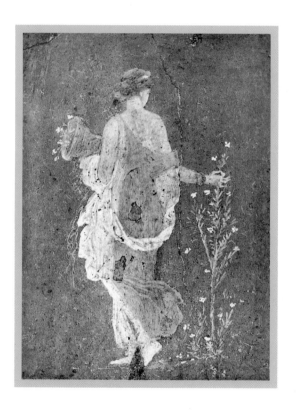

Bath Luxuries Shopping Guide

Abunda Life of America
P.O. Box 151
Avon by the Sea, NJ 07762
(201) 775-7575
Essential oils, luxury bath products

Aroma Therapy Products
P.O. Box 2354
Fair Oaks, CA 95628
(916) 965-7546
Essential oils

Aroma Vera
2728 South Robertson Boulevard
Los Angeles, CA 90034
(213) 280-0407
Essential oils

Aubrey Organics Bath Oils
4419 North Manhattan Avenue
Tampa, FL 33614
800-237-4270
Luxury bath products

Aveda
509 Madison Avenue
New York, NY 10022
(212) 832-2416
Essential oils, luxury bath products

Barney's New York
106 Seventh Avenue
New York, NY 10011
(212) 929-9000
Luxury bath products

John Bell & Croyden
Department A6 Mo
52-54 Wigmore Street
London W.I., England
44-71-935-5555
Essential oils

Belle Star, Inc.
23151 Alcalde, #C4
Laguna Hills, CA 92653
800-442-7827
Essential oils, luxury bath products

The Body Shop
1341 Seventh Street
Berkeley, CA 94710
(415) 524-0360
Essential oils, luxury bath products

The Body Shop International Ltd
Hawthorn Road
Little Hampton, West Sussex BN17
  7LR, England
44 (0903) 726-250
Luxury bath products, essential oils

H. Bronnley & Co. Ltd
10 Conduit Street
London W1R 0BR, England
44-71-629-8711
Luxury bath products

Capriland's Herb Farm
Silver Street
North Coventry, CT 06238
(203) 742-7244
Essential oils, dried herbs

Caswell-Massey Company
111 Eighth Avenue
New York, NY 10011
(212) 620-0900
Essential oils, luxury bath products

Chambers
Mail Order Department
P.O. Box 7841
San Francisco, CA 94120-7841
(415) 421-3277
Luxury bath products

Cherchez
862 Lexington Avenue
New York, NY 10021
(212) 620-0900
Essential oils, dried herbs

Crabtree & Evelyn Ltd
6 Kensington Church Street
London W8 2PD, England
44-71-937-9335
Essential oils, luxury bath products

Crabtree & Evelyn Ltd
Masonville Place
London, Ontario, Canada N6E 1R6
(519) 660-6601
Essential oils, luxury bath products

Crabtree & Evelyn Ltd
175 bd Saint-Germain
Paris, France
33-1-45-44-68-76
Essential oils, luxury bath products

Crabtree & Evelyn Ltd
30 East 67th Street
New York, NY 10028
(212) 734-1108
Essential oils, luxury bath products

Culpeper Ltd
21 Bruton Street
London W1X 7DA, England
44-71-499-2406
Essential oils, dried herbs

Czech & Speake
39c Jermyn Street
London SW1 6JH, England
44-71-439-0216
Essential oils, luxury bath products

The Essential Oil Co.
P.O. Box 88
Sandy, OR 97055
(503) 695-2400
Essential oils

Farmaceutica de Santa Maria Novella
Via della Scala, 16
50123, Florence, Italy
Essential oils, luxury bath products

Floris
89 Jermyn Street
London SW1 6JH, England
44-71-930-2885
Essential oils, luxury bath products

Floris
703 Madison Avenue
New York, NY 10021
(212) 935-9100
Essential oils, luxury bath products

Green Mountain Herbs Ltd
P.O. Box 2369
Boulder, CO 80306
800-525-2696
Essential oils, dried herbs

Dr. Hauschka Cosmetics, Inc.
Wala-Heitmittel GMBH
D-7325 Eckwalder, Bad Boll,
  Germany
Luxury bath products

Hove Parfumeur
723 Toulouse Street
New Orleans, LA 70130
(504) 525-7827
Essential oils, luxury bath products

Kiehl's Pharmacy
109 Third Avenue
New York, NY 10003
(212) 475-3400
Essential oils, dried herbs

Madini Oils
68F Tinker Street
Woodstock, NY 12498
(914) 679-7647
Essential oils

Maison Naturelle USA, Inc.
P.O. Box 730
Pine Brook, NJ 07058
(201) 882-1305
Luxury bath products

D. Napier & Sons
17 Bristol Place
Edinburgh, EHI, Scotland
44-31-225-5542
Dried herbs

Original Swiss Aromatics
P.O. Box 606
San Rafael, CA 94915
(415) 459-3998
Essential oils

Penhaligon's
41 Wellington Street
London WC2, England
44-71-836-2150
Luxury bath products

Ra-Bob International
320 Hillsdale Drive
Wichita, KS 67230
(316) 733-0904
Essential oils

Repêchage
212 Fifth Avenue
New York, NY 10010
(212) 532-2855
Luxury bath products

The Secret Garden
70 Westow Street
London SE19, England
44-71-771-8200

Self-Care Catalog
349 Healdsburg Avenue
Healdsburg, CA 95448
800-345-3371
Luxury bath products

Uncommon Scents, Inc.
555 High Street
Eugene, OR 97401
(503) 345-0952
Essential oils, luxury bath products

Victoria's Secret
Catalogue Division, North American
   Office
P.O. Box 16589
Columbus, OH 43216-6589
800-437-4438
Luxury bath products

Weleda, Inc.
841 South Main Street
Spring Valley, NY 10977
(914) 356-4134
Luxury bath products, dried herbs

Grateful acknowledgment is made for permission to reproduce
the following works of art:

Page 10: *My Sweet Rose* by John William Waterhouse, Roy
Miles Gallery, 29 Bruton Street, London, W1 / Bridgeman Art
Library, London.

Page 17: *The Birth of Venus* by Sandro Botticelli, Uffizi
Gallery, Scala/Art Resource.

Page 20: *Sunlight* by Frank W. Benson, © 1990 Indianapolis
Museum of Art, John Herron Fund.

Page 27: *Bather Arranging Her Hair* by Auguste Renoir,
National Gallery of Art, Washington, D.C., Chester Dale
Collection.

Page 30: *Woman on the Waves* by Paul Gauguin, The
Cleveland Museum of Art, Gift of Mr. and Mrs. William
Powell Jones, 78.63.

Page 37: *The Mirror* by Robert Reid, National Museum of
American Art, Smithsonian Institution, Gift of William T.
Evans.

Page 40: *Summer* by Sir Edward Burne-Jones, Roy Miles
Gallery, 29 Bruton Street, London, W1 / Bridgeman Art
Library, London.

Page 47: *The White Girl* by James McNeill Whistler, National
Gallery of Art, Washington, D.C., Harris Whittemore
Collection.

Page 50: *The Daydream* by Dante Gabriel Rossetti, by
permission of the Board of Trustees of the Victoria & Albert
Museum.

Page 57: *The Violet Kimono* by Robert Reid, National Museum
of American Art, Smithsonian Institution, Gift of John
Gellatly.

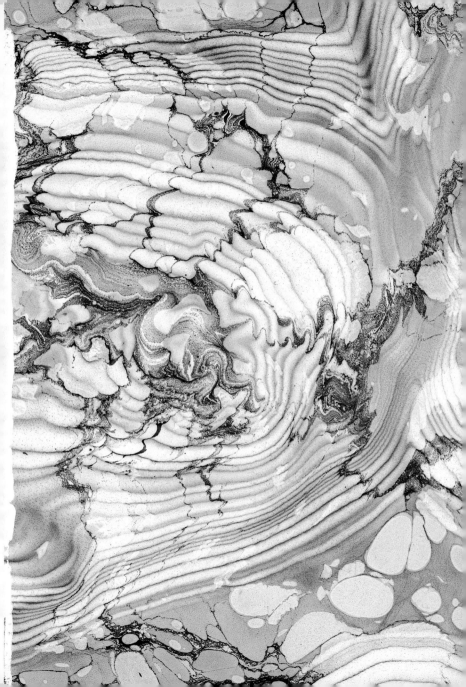

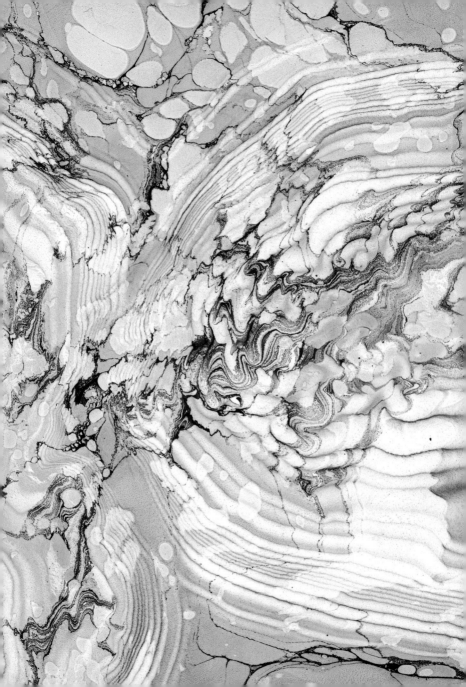